Dieting Vs. Weight Loss
Breaking The Habits
By: Dan Ouellette

ISBN: 978-1508543879

Growing up I was always a skinny kid. Even when I went into the Army at eighteen, I only weighed 110 pounds. I packed on the weight while I was in there though. (That picture to the right is me at 19. Before my weight gain.) When I got out, I was a whopping 136 pounds.

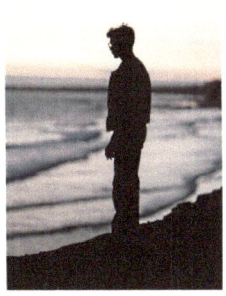

The majority of the weight I gained back then was muscle, but from then on it was all down hill. (Well, not really... My weight went up and down and up and down over the years. I would try watching what I ate for a few weeks and then give it up when I couldn't tolerate the starving any longer, or when someone had a birthday and the cake and ice cream looked too tempting.

Then it all changed. At 49 years old, and "slightly" over 200 pounds, I decided enough was enough. I had already tried making some changes to my diet, but not the ones that really mattered. I tried eating low-fat, low calorie, low carb, etc... But that didn't change a thing. So I decided to go with my gut instincts and drop all of the "diet fad" stuff. I even went against my doctor's advice.

I switched back to real butter. I went back to real milk. I paid the extra money and bought peanut oil instead of vegetable oil. If the package indicated it was low anything, I avoided it like the plague... Why would I choose to eat something that has been altered? When natural substances are removed from a product, man-made chemicals or other ingredients are added to make up for the flavor or consistency. Your body doesn't know how to process these ingredients. You are just sabotaging your diet because you think you are eating healthier, but you're not.
Keep in mind that your body was designed to process natural fats, natural sugars, natural salts, and other natural ingredients. So why substitute natural with man-made? It doesn't make sense to me...

I like to cook, so my decision was a simple one. I started making more of my own meals. I stopped buying prepackaged things like hamburger helper (which I love), and other boxed foods. Instead, I bought a bag of potatoes, a bag of white rice, spaghetti noodles, egg noodles, macaroni noodles, canned veggies, frozen veggies, some fresh veggies, bread, tortillas, and plain meats like pork chops, chicken (and I am talking with the skin on), ground beef, sausage, ham steaks, etc.

Most diets will tell you to stop eating things like pasta, potatoes, eggs, chips, cookies, brownies, cakes, pastries, etc... But why deprive yourself of any of that stuff? You don't have to. But what you have to do is know where the limit is. (Keep in mind that those things are still processed and do contain man-made ingredients.) For a healthier alternative, you could always try baking treats from scratch. A home-made cake, brownies, and cookies are healthier than pre-made / pre-packaged ones from the store.

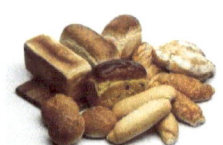 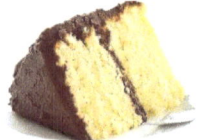 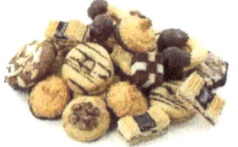

If your diet plan forbids you from eating these, then you're on the wrong plan!!!

Let's face it, you love food. Who doesn't? I'll admit it; I love food. I love to eat. I often start thinking about my next meal before I even finish the one I'm on. I even plan my vacation itinerary around the restaurants I want to go to when I go home for a visit.

HOME COOKING

Now if you are saying you hate cooking, well that's too bad. Learn to accept the fact that you need to cook your own meals and move on. It doesn't take much time to throw a meal into the crockpot. I have cooked things like meatloaf, chinese pie (shepherd's pie) beef roast, pork roast, ribs, pasta sauces, etc in the crockpot. Make it even easier on yourself and create meals ahead of time in a gallon size ziplock bag and freeze them. At least then you know what's going into the bag and into your mouth.

Think about something for a moment... Who is really telling us what to eat and what is healthy for us? Our government? How many of them are skinny? No, it's the conglomerates that own businesses that make money off of man-made ingredients? They are the ones telling us what it healthy and what is not.

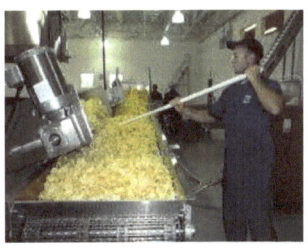

If you were to look around the world and look for the people with the lowest portion of overweight people, you will find that those people don't have easy access to fast foods, low-fat, low-calorie products. They don't need fad diets because they eat natural foods. Many countries ban man-made ingredients because they are bad for you.

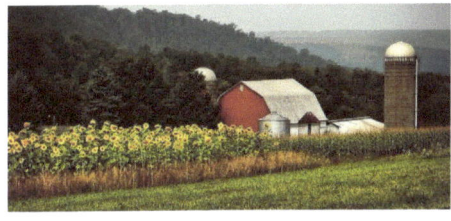

Think about the family that lives on a farm. They eat potatoes, meat, whole milk, real butter, eggs, vegetables, etc. How many overweight farmers do you know? Not many. They do work the farm, so they do get exercise, but they also don't eat as much pre-packaged foods that most Americans eat daily.

BAD HABITS ARE TAUGHT

If you are like me, when you were growing up you heard people say things like, "You better eat more or you'll be hungry in an hour.", or

"Don't eat that, we're eating in an hour." Wrong!!! You're hungry now, so eat something. Then in an hour you won't need to eat as much.

On another note, if you are nearing the end of your meal and you say something along the lines of "I ate too much", then guess what??? You ate too much.

We, as a population, have gone about demanding larger portions at restaurants and expecting more. Now that we have larger portions, we feel we have to eat everything on our plate or we are wasting it.

When I go to a restaurant, I try to minimize my bad habits. I will try to share my meal with someone. I will order from the appetizer section or the A-la-carte section. At a fast food restaurant, I will order the kid's meal. Or I will eat a portion and take the rest home for later. But on occasion, I will eat the whole thing...

One of the biggest downfalls for dieters is the buffet. But for me, that is one of the best places to go. There I get to eat a large variety of different foods all at once. The trick is, smaller portions. The drawback is that I don't get my money's worth at a buffet.

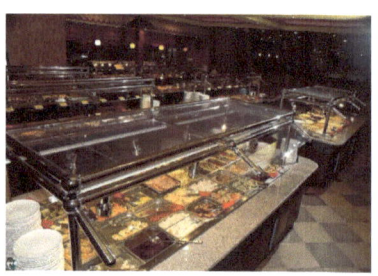

But at least I get to keep my weight in-check!

SO NOW YOU ARE ASKING "WHAT DO I EAT?"

Up to this point you've heard me tell you what to avoid. So now I am going to tell you what I typically eat.

BREAKFAST

A typical day for me when I get up, I either fry up or scramble a couple eggs. Throw in a couple

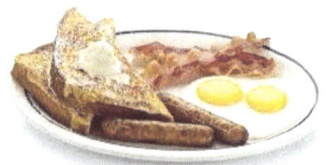

pieces of bacon, or half of a small ham steak, or if I have time I make a home made egg & muffin or two pieces of french toast complete with real butter and maple syrup. Another option is two sausage pinwheels and a little country gravy. As you can see, I don't shy away from the foods I love. But I don't over-indulge like I used to.

On weekends I might add homefries or hashbrowns to the mix as an added treat because I lost more weight than I expected that week. So when you add up a week's worth of weight loss, I could do better without the "weekend reward", but why not indulge a little. I did great all week long. I deserve a break.

But you might be thinking that there just isn't enough breakfast to keep you going until lunch. Well you're right. But that is the way you need to start thinking from now on.

You have to stop thinking about eating enough food to last you for four to six hours in-between meals.

Instead, you need to eat enough to last you 1 ½ to 2 hours.

When you start to get hungry again, eat something. If you like fruit, eat fruit. If you like peanut butter and jelly sandwich, then eat it. Personally, I like to snack on potatoes. It doesn't matter what kind of potatoes. That's up to you to decide. I might bake a potato in the microwave and add some butter. I might grab 8 saltines and 2 slices of cheese, or 8 Ritz crackers with peanut butter. Graham crackers and peanut butter is amazing too! Pop some popcorn in a brown sack and add some real butter. Throw a piece of ham, bologna, or turkey on a piece of bread with a little mustard or mayo. You can even throw a piece of lettuce and cheese on it too. It's just a snack so it shouldn't be a whole sandwich loaded up with the works.

Most, if not all diets tell you to limit potatoes. But I think they are all wrong. You shouldn't eliminate natural foods. You should only eat smaller portions. So stop thinking back to all of those other diets you were on.

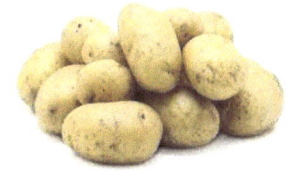

Potatoes are not bad for your diet. Trust me! They are very filling, but more important, they are very natural. You can even add a little bit of sour cream, butter, and cheese. But just add enough to flavor it. Remember, it isn't a meal, it's just a snack. And, you're supposed to be hungry again in 1 ½ to 2 hours.

LUNCH-TIME

Now before you know it, it's lunch time. You should be starting to feel a little hungry again and you planned ahead so you don't have to run off to a fast food place. You can either eat leftovers from the night before, or you can eat a sandwich, or just about anything else that comes to mind. Just do it in moderation.

While you are sitting there eating your lunch, your co-workers are in awe because they either brought in a three course meal, ran out to get a greasy burger, or they are loading up their huge salad with fat-free dressing. Won't they be surprised when you start shedding the pounds and they gave up on their diet again... They just don't understand why you are losing all this weight when all you do is eat all day long...

And that is the "secret" to this diet plan. Spread out your calorie intake throughout your day and your body begins to burn off those calories more evenly. You then get your metabolism back on track. That is when the weight really disappears.

This isn't a miracle diet. It is a way of life. And as soon as you train yourself to think correctly about your eating habits, you'll figure out just how much easier your life has become. Oh yeah, and you keep losing more weight along the way.

SIDE EFFECTS

We all know that with most actions comes a reaction. Eating right has some side effects. The main side-effect is your weight loss. But, there may also be another benefit that you'll begin to notice. You will probably become more regular. You might be wondering why or how. So let's figure this out...

You put the natural fats back into your diet. You know, the natural fats from real butter, real mayo or miracle whip, real milk, that delicious skin from the chicken that you ate last night. Or maybe it was from the peanut oil that you fried your food in last night. Either way, you reintroduced natural fats into your body and eliminated the fake stuff like vegetable oil and unnatural ingredients from those so-called diet foods.

Other side-effects to a better diet is less acne, better complexion, shinier hair, stronger fingernails, more energy, and a better night's sleep. Don't ask me why, it just happens. Now if I had formal training, I might be able to answer that question, but I don't. It just happens.

SOMETHING TO THINK ABOUT

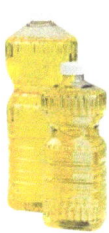

Name a vegetable that has natural oil in it... Go ahead. Name one... That's what I thought. You can't come up with even one example. Now go look at the label on a bottle of vegetable oil. Could you find even one vegetable listed in the ingredients? While you are looking at the label, describe what each of the ingredients are. (HINT: vegetable oil is not made from vegetables.)

Now grab that bottle of peanut oil and read the ingredients... There shouldn't be any question as to which oil you should be using. Now I know it is more expensive, but it is well worth the extra expense to have a more natural product touching your food.

Also, vegetable oils like canola, sunflower, cottonseed, safflower, etc raise your risk of cardiovascular disease compared to natural oils.

There is also another alternative to processes oils. You can look for real lard. You can't get more natural than that. But make sure it is real lard and not that man-made fake stuff made to look like lard. If you are wondering why I am mentioning real lard when it has been deemed so unhealthy, let me ask you this... Why has the number of incidents of clogged arteries increased since the invention of vegetable oil? The answer is because vegetable oil is not natural. Nothing in vegetable oil is natural. So why would you want to put that in your body?

Think about shortening and margarine for a moment. They have to do things and add things to those two items in order to make them look the way they do or no one would buy them. They have to hold their shape and/or consistency at and above room temperature for a period of time. So what do you think happens to that stuff in your body?

DINNER

I know I got off track and never mentioned dinner. That is usually the hardest meal if you are in a relationship or have kids. I say that because your partner was probably raised by heathens who made him or her eat three big meals a day full of processed foods or they hated to cook and brought home fast food most every night. (Unless of course you lucked out and they were raised on a farm.) But regardless, stick to your plan and they will eventually see that once again, you were right and they were wrong.

Now your kids are another matter all together. You have total control over them and what they eat. (If not, then you have parenting issues that I will cover in my next book.) So before it's too late, drop your old habits and start teaching them how to eat properly. They will thank you when they get older!

I went online to pull a picture to add to this section and when I typed in "dinner plate" every last one of the over 1,000 photos I saw had too much food on the plate. So instead of showing you an unrealistic picture, we'll just for-go the image.

"POPULAR" DIET PLANS

I wasn't going to mention them, but the more I thought about it the more I began leaning towards including it. So here it is... There are at least two popular weight-loss programs that advertise on television where you buy their prepackaged meals for up to a month at a time.

Don't waste your money. No matter who you are, you will be hungry. One group of you will be hungry because the portions are too small and you don't have enough "snacks" to fill the gaps. The other group will be hungry because many of those meals are just plain nasty and you refuse to eat the whole portion.

The concept is correct. Portion control is the key. But the execution and quality just isn't there. How can you be satisfied when the food just doesn't satisfy? Plus, read the ingredients list. What exactly are they forcing you to put into your body under the guise of nutritional diet food?

I hate to mention this too because I love her as an actress, but how many times does she have to balloon up and slim down before she realizes what she is doing wrong? You know who I mean!

So take my advice or not, but please stay as far away from that stuff as possible.

MEAL & SNACK OPTIONS

The next section outlines some food options, but those options are in no way everything that you can and should eat. They are just some of the meals and snacks I like and the stuff that helped me lose my weight. So pick and choose the things you like and come up with your own healthy portions of the foods you love. If you do that and stick to this plan, you will see just how easy it is to lose and then maintain your weight.

I know it may be hard for you to wrap your head around many of the things I talked about here, but forget what you read about with all of those fad diets you've tried in the past, because honestly, this isn't a diet. It is a way of living. If you follow this advice, you should never be left hungry. You should never be left craving something you can't eat. And you will never have to think about dieting again.

So give it 30 days and see what happens.

FOOD IDEAS

Now I know you are going to look at some of the items I use and say things like: "That's loaded with salt.", or "That's not all natural.", or whatever else you can think of... But there are times where I cheat and use items out of convenience. And that's fine to do as long as you use those items sparingly. I'm talking about gravy mixes, salad dressings, jellies and jams, and other such condiments. If you can make them home made, then all the more power to you! I'm just a bit lazy about some things...

Breakfast Ideas

I like orange juice, but you can drink whatever you want with your breakfast. Coffee, tea, milk, whatever. But stay away from artificial sweeteners. They are not natural and should not be in your routine.

2 eggs (any style) - 1 pc toast w/butter – 2 pc bacon

2 eggs (scrambled & fried) – pc cheese – w/mayo – on 2 pc bread

1 biscuit – 1 sausage cut up – 1/2 cup country gravy – 1 fried egg

2 -3 sausage pinwheels – 2 tbls country gravy (optional)

2 egg omelet – ½ cup meat – ¼ cup cheese – any veggies you want to add

1 cup fried potatoes – 1 sausage – 1 egg – sprinkle of cheese

Bowl of cereal with whole milk (I like Frosted Flakes or Coco Puffs)

1 toast – ½ S.O.S. – 1 egg

1 breakfast burrito with bacon, egg, cheese, & potatoes

1 home made egg, ham & cheese on a muffin

Now these are my choices. You can create your own. Just keep the portion size within reason. Now I know that you might be worried that you don't have time to make this stuff in the morning. That's fine. Make it the night before. Or make a bunch of the stuff on

Sunday. What I do is buy the biggest box of small and large generic ziplock bags and make enough meals for Monday thru Thursday or Friday. You can fry up eggs for fried egg sandwiches, or a batch of sausage gravy, scrambled eggs, bacon, fried potatoes, breakfast burritos, etc. Just separate everything out to one portion meals per baggie. Zap them in the microwave and throw it together. You can even freeze any of these items for a few weeks if need be. If I have more than I need, I set them aside for snacks or lunches. Who doesn't like breakfast for lunch or dinner?

Lunches

Lunches can be another challenge at first, but once you get on a roll, it should come much easier. I have found that one of the easiest ways of making my lunches is to use what I had for dinner the night before. Made a roast? Slice it up for a sandwich the next day. Extra pork chops? They also make a great sandwich. There are many options, but I tend to like leftovers the next day. They always seem to taste better when reheated.

Some of the things I make special for lunches include:
ham salad, chicken salad, egg salad, cucumber salad, fried bologna sandwich, grilled ham & cheese, grilled bologna and cheese, mashed potato sandwich, cucumber sandwich, 2 hotdogs w/bun, etc...

If I want something hot, I like to make some home made chicken or pork fried rice or lo mein. I say home made because it is pretty easy and I put in what I like. I also make enough that I can snack on it for a week.

Dinners
Crockpot, crockpot, crockpot. Get to know your crockpot intimately. There are websites dedicated to crockpot recipes. All I ask that you keep in mind is to keep as close to natural ingredients as possible. You can cook so many things in a crockpot, but I will caution you when it comes to spaghetti sauce, it tends to burn if you aren't there to stir it.

1 inch thick Meatloaf – 1 baked potato w/butter – veggie – slice of buttered bread

1 porkchop – fried or baked seasoned potatoes – veggie

1 cup beef tips w/gravy - 1 cup rice or egg noodles - veggie

1 hand full pasta – 2-4 meatballs – 1 cup sauce – 1 slice garlic bread

3-4 hand breaded chicken tenders – hand full french fries – lots of ketchup!!!

1 ½ - 2 cups fried kielbasa & fried potatoes (I fry them together with onions using butter)

Taco salad (ground beef, refried bean, cheese, lettuce, tomatoes, sour cream, taco sauce)
1 cup ground beef (fried) w/brown gravy – 1 cup rice – veggies – slice bread w/butter

1 baked chicken breast w/skin – 1 cup of rice-a-roni – veggie

2 beef or chicken fajitas w/small tortilla – lettuce – tomatoes – sour cream – cheese – salsa

2 cups albondigas soup (meatball soup) – 4-5 tortilla chips crushed on top

2 cups chili w/cornbread – ¼ cup cheese

4" x 4" square shepherd's pie – 1 slice of butter bread

½ ham steak – 1 cup scalloped potatoes – veggie

Meatball sandwich (use a potato bun hot dog roll) w/6 meatballs – ¼ cup mozzarella cheese

1 cup sliced pork – 1 cup rice-a-roni - veggies
Again, anything you chose to make should work with this. Just use reasonable portions. Keep in mind that this isn't the last meal of the day either. You still have time for a snack or two before going to bed. One of the things I like to have at night is a peanut butter and jam sandwich. I had read that peanut butter late in the evening helps raise your metabolism while you sleep. Not sure how true that is, but

I love peanut butter and jam/jelly, so what the hell...

Snacks
Snacks can be virtually anything you want. Eat a couple cookies, or a twinkie. Pop a batch of popcorn and add butter to taste (do not buy prepackaged microwave popcorn though) Instead, buy an air popper or use a ¼ cup of kernels in a brown paper lunch bag in the microwave. It tastes better and not loaded with chemicals.

2 – 4 cookies, 1 small bag of chips, 2 slices cheese & 8 saltines, popcorn, ½ cheese crisp w/salsa, hand full of pretzels, sliced apple, orange, banana, grapes, etc...

One thing I did not do over the past four months was deprive myself of any type of food that I wanted. That included Ho-Ho's, Snickers, Ben & Jerry's, Burger King's original chicken sandwich, KFC', etc... But when I chose to eat any of those items, I knew I was either not going to lose as much weight during that week or I would chose better options on the other days that week.

<u>CHECKING YOUR WEIGHT</u>

I know many diets tell you not to weigh yourself but maybe once a week or so. I say screw that... But, I will say the first thing you need to do is weigh yourself before you begin. Write down that weight somewhere and then don't step on the scale again for the first three weeks. Whenever you change the way you eat, your weight will go up and down. You don't want to be discouraged right at the

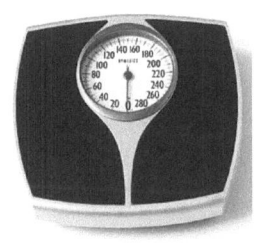

beginning. But after those first three weeks, then go ahead and step on that scale every morning. That way you see what yesterday's eating habits did for you. As each day goes by and you see that you lost a pound or gained a pound, think about the foods you ate, the quantity you ate per setting, and make an adjustment. (But DO NOT make adjustments that will cause you to starve yourself.)

Keep in mind, if 2 hours have passed and you're not hungry, you ate too much at your last meal!

EXCURSIONS & VACATIONS

I also want to point out that during those four months that I lost the weight, I went home to Maine. I figured when I was there I would need to indulge in the types of food you can only get back home. So I knew I would be eating lobster, fried clams, the local hamburger joint, my favorite pizza, clam cakes, etc. And I most certainly did eat every last one of those items. But I also made the right choices. I split my meal with a family member. Not only did we both save money, we both kept our portion sizes reasonable. I think we were the only two people not complaining about eating too much when we sat around the table chatting after-wards. And guess what... A couple hours later, we indulged ourselves with an ice cream. I ended up losing weight even while on vacation and I got to eat all of my favorite foods!

So it isn't that hard. Just stop thinking like a dieter and start changing the way you look at food, portion sized, designated meal times, and mis-information being fed to you by so-called experts. Oh, by-the-way, I am not a nutritionist, I am not a dietitian, I am not a representative of a major anything, I am just a person who lost thirty-five pounds enjoying all the foods I love.

UNORTHODOX COMPARISON

I just had another thought... I know this may seem completely off-topic, but I had a ten year old dog when I was given a second dog. I had always left the dry dog food out where they could get to it when they wanted. The 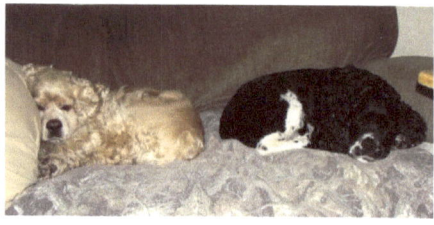 first dog grew up like that and never over-ate. The second dog wasn't used to that. And for the first couple of weeks, he would stand in front of the bowl and eat non-stop. At least until the first dog would force him out of the way.

After the first two weeks and putting on quite a few pounds, he realized that there was always food available and he stopped gorging. From then on, he would go eat a few bites throughout the day and walk away. He started losing weight within a week or two and he became slimmed down to a normal weight within a couple of months.

So, while I am not trying to compare anyone to a dog, what I am saying here is that if you just eat enough food to maintain your comfort, you will find the perfect balance and the perfect portion size.

PERSONAL RESPONSIBILITY

I am a strong believe of personal responsibility, but I also know that in this case it isn't all your fault. Your parents probably made you clean your plate before getting up from the table, you might have been forced into believing there were starving children in some third-world country that would gladly eat the food you left on your plate if you could get it to them, grandparents probably kept offering you food the whole time you were visiting them, restaurants determined what a portion size should be, fast food places had the option to super-size, nutritionist told you what to eat and what not to eat, diet books told you to cut out the wrong foods, corporations told you to eat low-fat, low-sugar, low-carb, low calorie this and low calorie that. And look at us now. We are a nation of obese people who live to eat instead eating to live.

So before you go any further into this, get up, go over to your bookcase, pull out every last one of your diet books, and throw them in the trash or fireplace. Or, if you're part of the electronic generation, delete that app off your phone or trash that ebook you bought. You will never need any of them again.

You are now responsible for your own eating habits and you will lose weight without starving!

IN CONCLUSION

This book isn't going to lay out your menu. That is something you need to do. But I encourage you to take the time to think about the foods you like to eat and think about how you can remove most of the artificial ingredients and go back to the more natural ingredients. If the label has a whole bunch of ingredients and you can't pronounce many of them, then think about an alternative. If it's something you really want, then go ahead and use it, but make adjustments elsewhere when you can.

I wish you the best of luck with your new way of thinking and eating. If enough people realize where we have been making our mistakes, then maybe the next generations after us will have a better understanding of proper nutrition and proper eating habits!

EXERCISE

I almost forgot... I hate exercising, so I don't... But what I do instead is I park further away from the entrance to the grocery store, or the mall and walk. Instead of circling the parking lot five or six times, I park anywhere I can find and walk. I also have a habit on getting all the way to the other end of the grocery store and realize the other item I needed is clear on the other end. Once you go back and forth across the store enough times, you could have put in a good mile or even two if you are as scatter-brained as I am in a grocery store.

The other thing I do, which may sound a bit silly, but I enjoy it... I lock my office door (at home) put on my headphones, and crank the dance music, and dance for about four or five, sometimes six songs. I don't really dance though. I more or less stretch to the beat of the music. If you think about it, four or five songs at three to four minutes each comes to about twelve minutes on the low end up to about thirty minutes on the high end. That wasn't exercise that was having fun for less than thirty minutes. Just make sure the webcam on your computer is unplugged and the curtains are drawn or you might end up on youtube.com

GOOD LUCK!

Some of my easy Recipes

BBQ Chicken Wings

INGREDIENTS:

20	each	chicken wings
1	jar	blackberry jam (or) orange marmalade
1	jar	barbecue sauce (any flavor)

DIRECTIONS:

In a large bowl, mix 1/2 jar jam to full jar bbq sauce. Dump in wings and mix well. Place in crockpot on low for 6-8 hours. Stir and serve.

Country Fried Potatoes

INGREDIENTS:

2-3	lg	potatoes (thin sliced)
1	ea	onion (sliced or chopped)
1	tsp	garlic (adjust for your taste)
1	tbsp	real butter

DIRECTIONS:

Mix everything in a bowl or ziplock and mix well. Pour into frying pan and cook on med-low 20-25 min. Flip over and cook another 20-25 min.

Home-Fries

INGREDIENTS:

2-3	lg	potatoes (cubed, boiled, & refrigerated overnight)
1	ea	onion (sliced)
2	tbsp	real butter
		salt & pepper (to taste)

DIRECTIONS:

Mix everything in a frying pan and cook on med-high until potatoes are crispy and browned

Three Envelope Roast

INGREDIENTS:

3	lb	beef roast (such as chuck roast)
1	env	dry Italian salad dressing mix
1	env	dry ranch salad dressing mix
1	env	dry brown gravy mix
2	cups	water

DIRECTIONS:

Mix water & seasoning together. Put everything into crockpot.
Cook on high 4 hrs (or) low 8 hrs.

Albondigas Soup

INGREDIENTS:

30	ea	italian meatballs	2	cups	picante sauce or salsa
6	cups	water	6	ea	beef bullion cubes
1	can	green beans (cut)	6	ea	chicken bullion
1	ea	onion (chopped)	2	ea	tomatoes (cubed)
1	cup	frozen peas	1	can	carrots (cut)
2	ea	potato (cubed)	1	tsp	onion powder
1	tsp	chili powder	1	tsp	season salt
1	tsp	crushed red peppers	1	tbls	chives (freeze dried ok)
1	tsp	chipotle seasoning			

DIRECTIONS:

Place in stew pot and simmer 2 hours.

Brown Sugar Syrup

INGREDIENTS:

2	cups	brown sugar	1/2	tsp	vanilla extract
1	cup	water	1	stk	real butter

DIRECTIONS:

Heat brown sugar & water on med heat until bubbling. Simmer 4
min then stir in butter until dissolved. Take off heat and stir in
vanilla. Cool 5 min, then pour into serving container.
(Store in fridge up to 3 months)

Crockpot Chex Mix

INGREDIENTS:

1/4	stk	butter	4	tsp	worcestershire sauce
1	tsp	salt	1	tsp	garlic powder
1/2	tsp	onion powder	1/4	tsp	sugar
3	cups	wheat, rice, & corn chex cereal			
1	cup	peanuts	1	cup	pretzels

DIRECTIONS:

Dissolve spices in butter, mix everything and place in crockpot.
Cook on low for 2.5 hrs, stir every 30 min.

Chinese Pie

INGREDIENTS:

1	lb	ground beef	1	med	onion (chopped)
2	cans	whole kernel corn	2	cans	cream-style corn
8	cups	mashed potatoes			

(If you prefer green beans, make a packet of brown gravy and pour over meat)

DIRECTIONS:

Brown beef & onions, place in 9x9 casserole dish. Mix corn and
pour over top. Layer mashed potatoes on top. Bake at 350 for
30 minutes.

Chicken Tenders

INGREDIENTS:

2	ea	breasts	2	ea	egg
1	cup	italian bread crumbs	1	cup	milk

DIRECTIONS:

Mix egg & milk. Cut chicken into strips, mix into egg. Pull one out
at a time and shake in bread crumbs until coated. Deep fry pieces
in peanut oil until golden brown. (1 - 1 1/2 minutes usually)

Crockpot Chicken & Dumplings

INGREDIENTS:

4	ea	chicken breast (cubed)	2	tbls	real butter
2	cans	cream of chicken soup	1	ea	onion (chopped)
3		tubes biscuit dough	1	can	carrots (drained)
1	can	green beans (drained)	3	cans	chicken broth
1	tsp	minced garlic			

DIRECTIONS:

Mix everything but dough in crockpot. Cook on high for 4-5 hrs. Cut each biscuit dough into 4 pcs & stir into crockpot. Cook for 2 hrs longer.

Brisket & Cabbage

INGREDIENTS:

1	pkg	pre-cooked brisket	1	lg	cabbage (sliced)
1	stk	real butter	1	lg	onion (chopped)

DIRECTIONS:

Place everything in an electric frying pan or skillet. Cook on med until onions & cabbage are softened. Turn heat to med-high and brown to your liking.

Mini Quiches

INGREDIENTS:

6	ea	eggs	3/4	cup	whole milk
2	ea	sausage links (cooked)	4	pcs	bacon (cooked)
1/2	tsp	dry mustard	1/2	tsp	onion powder
1/2	tsp	dried chives	1	cup	shredded cheese

DIRECTIONS:

Spray pan with Pam. Mix eggs with spices. Divide into 12 slot muffin pan. Sprinkle some cheese then sausage & bacon pcs into each slot. Sprinkle cheese again & then chives. Bake on 350 for 25 min. (Lasts 4-5 days in fridge)

Sausage Pinwheels

INGREDIENTS:

1   pkg   breakfast sausage roll

1   pkg   crescent roll dough

1   pkg   country gravy

DIRECTIONS:

Roll out the dough. Break up and spread the uncooked sausage onto the dough. Roll up and slice 1/2 inch thick circles. Place on cookie sheet & bake on 350 for 20-25 min. (Until browned) Serve with gravy.

Better Popcorn

INGREDIENTS:

1/4   cup   popcorn kernels   1   tbsp   real butter

1   ea   brown lunch bag

DIRECTIONS:

Melt the butter in microwave bowl, set aside. Pour popcorn into bag and microwave for 1 1/2 - 2 1/2 min or until popping stops (Each microwave is different) Pour butter & salt into bag and shake. Pour into bowl & serve.

No-Mess Bacon

INGREDIENTS:

1-2   lb   bacon

1   ea   deep fryer

DIRECTIONS:

Heat deep fryer to highest setting. Place 5-6 pcs of bacon into oil. Cook 1-2 minutes slowly stirring. Remove when it looks almost done and place onto 3-4 layers of paper towels to drain. Reduce time if too crispy. Can store for a week in fridge.

Baked Chicken Wings

INGREDIENTS:

1	bag	chicken wings (thawed)	1	ea	bbq sauce
1	jar	orange marmalade			

DIRECTIONS:

Mix bbq sauce & marmalade in bowl. Mix in chicken & place in fridge overnight. Remove wings & place on baking pan. Bake 1 hr on 350 degrees.

Sausage & Potatoes

INGREDIENTS:

1	lb	sausage or kilbasa	2	lg	potatoes (cubed)
1	ea	onion (sliced)	2	tbsp	real butter

salt & pepper to taste

DIRECTIONS:

Saute all on med in a skillet until potatoes are softened. Turn heat to med-high and fry until browned.

Beef Tips & Gravy

INGREDIENTS:

2	lbs	stew beef	1	ea	onion (sliced)
1	cup	water	3	pkg	brown gravy mix
1	tsp	minced garlic	1	sm	sour cream

DIRECTIONS:

Cook beef, onion, garlic, and water in crockpot on low for 6-8 hrs. When finished, make gravy per pkg. Mix gravy & sour cream into crockpot. Serve over egg noodles or rice.